The Body The Blood The Bug

By RL Lane

ISBN: 1523255889
ISBN-13: 978-1523255887

The body the blood the bug...

You only have one
The body
It started dying the minute you were born

The blood
stays in it while the heart pumps life through it
Then it goes
The blood comes out

Then it goes
Down in the ground
Or in a fire to ashes...

I know a lot of people
Who like to forget
You only have one body

It doesn't go with you when you die
You die
No matter how much you wish you hope you pray

The strongest willed
Succumb at the end
The blood comes out

When life is no more
No more
Your money can't bring it back

Your money can't bring you back…

These words are they harsh?
They should be
When will you listen?
When will you let it rest?
20 is not 30 is not 40 is not 50...
Treat your body with respect the older it gets

Listen to it when it is hungry
When it is thirsty
When it is cold
When it is tired

Give it food
Give it water
Give it shelter
Give it rest

Like the innkeeper gave Mary and the donkey
For the baby to be born…

Prayers don't work
Let me be 20
Prayers don't work
Please stop the time

Prayers only work
On the things that are possible

They can make miracles
But not the miracle of age

You can hide the age
Cover it with a mask
But it is still below it
Wondering why you can't see it…

Will you just look one day
In the mirror at night
And see the wrinkle
And believe your fate?
Toy were...you were born to die
Toy...you were given toys as a child
To help you learn
Did they forget to teach you how life really works?

So I wrote this book
A simple reminder
Not to make you sad
But to hell…help you to understand
Whether you believe in heaven or hell

You are not indestructible
No matter how much you want to be
Why would you beat up your body?
The only one that you have
Can't you learn from the past?

Then I saw her
A tall black woman
Her hair was not long
No glasses
She was wearing pants
Her hands were in her pockets
Somehow she helps my ex-husband
This book was written for my brother
But maybe it's for him too

Really it's for every man and buy...boy
Every woman and girl
To remember
You can't buy time
And your body gets old
As your time runs out…

Treat it with respect
Don't make it carry around the extra weight
Don't make it run on caffeine and no sleep

Maybe the innkeeper just wanted to help the donkey
Let the old girl rest
Give her a drink
Maybe he loved those old gray donkeys
And the sound...he used to love to hear the sound they made

The bug
What about the bug?
It came around when I was writing this book

It was huge
The biggest bug I have ever seen
It got in my house and then it disappeared
I tried to find it because I knew…

I found it the next morning
Dead in a corner
Upside-down lying on its back
It made me sad because I would have liked to save it
If I could have caught it I would have put it back outside
Because I knew…

It was in the kitchen and then it just disappeared
I thought maybe it had crawled in a cupboard
I went to bed
I was afraid I would wake up and it would be staring me in the face…

Like age. I will wake up one day and it will stare me in the face as I look into the mirror…

Will it be too late?
Like it was for the bug
Will I listen before it is too late?

The bug
It was just a cricket
They symbolize good luck and protection
Everyone can use good luck
And protection
This was a giant cricket
Would it have meant a lot of good luck
And protection?

I couldn't save it
Did I try hard enough?
It was just a bug you say
Is that what you always say?

Minimize the important to suit your needs
Just one more cigarette
Just one more drink
Just one more doughnut…

Or should it be
Just
One more lap
Just
One more fight
Just
One more night
Just
One more morning
Just…

Remember the bug
Every morning you awake
He couldn't be saved
But if you are still reading…

You can be…

About the Author and Illustrator

RL Lane has published the EcarreT series and a collection of short stories featuring the illustrations, along with the children's books "G" and "How to Catch a Goast". The series begins with "Chapel Street Signs"…

...unexplained connections that challenge us to beli ve. A woman, a Dad a Doctor, a cat and mouse, a horse and tale tell their stories. "Do you beli ve in spirits?" I asked my friend. "Well look", he said, "I believe there are things that cannot be explained..." Oh. Plus, hear ov a Mom's battle with her struggle to connect to the woman...her little girl.

Welcome to EcarreT...a world
Where everyone cares
Why did I have to create it in...

A fiction fantasy world?

You may already know why, but you will see regardless of what you believe as a girl's journey of love and faith on her "Touring Machine" take her on the best journey of her mundane life. A life well on its way takes a turn in a direction that could've never been seen or even dreamed...

The author can be contacted at:

readrllane@gmail.com
www.Amazon.com/author/readrllane

Twitter.com/readrllane

Books by RL Lane

EcarreT Series:

Chapel Street Signs
secret Life OV an antE
Sri Town
Which of EcarreT

Hand of Heven

Bells to Believe

Short Stories:

Mon Treal, The Odd Cod, The Half Day, No Gift for Greed, Aunt Elm & Uncle
Poc, What Would Caitlin Wear, The Bag of Scribbles, Mr. Uraly's Italy, A not G,
Johnni and Georg, A Cup of Butter, The Walk of a THOUSAND Moods, Storm
Window, The Rugs, Cones of Ice Crème, Angel-A, The Art of Sri Town, Under
Water, The Dinner Party, The Vault, No Lines to Erase, Rock of Snow, Spilled
Sugar, A Rug and a Bag, Polka Dot Rain Boots, The Stations, The Copper Head,
No Cheese, Mr. Storior

Children's:

G

How to Catch a Goast

A-Me

Coming Soon

Bubble ov lOVe

www.ingramcontent.com/pod-product-compliance
Lightning Source LLC
Chambersburg PA
CBHW081546280526
45788CB00010B/3375